Proven Lifestyle, Keto Diet and Paleo Formula for Reversing Type 2 Diabetes

Simplified Self Help Guide on Fruits and Food for Normal Blood Sugar

by

Arnold Bridge M.D

Dedication

For Christiana, with love!

Acknowledgements

My esteem regards to my colleagues and equally Diabetes patients who gave relevant hints in the preparation of this book.

Table of Contents

CHAPTER ONE

1.0 Diabetes: The Basics

Diabetes (Diabetes mellitus) is a common chronic medical condition that affects the way the human body handles glucose, a kind of sugar, in the blood, and the most prevalent of which is Type 2. The United States Center for Disease Control and Prevention report that in the United States, over 29 million people have diabetes, ie. 9.3 percent of the population. It has a powerful effect on the heart with resultant cardiovascular disease, being heart disease and stroke, and can also lead to complications during pregnancy. Prediabetes on the other hand is a condition where the blood glucose is not normal, but not high enough to be tagged- diabetes. Of note, hormone insulin helps move sugar from the blood into human cells, which are where the sugar is used for energy. In particular, for Type 2 Diabetes, the body cells are unable to respond to insulin as well as they should and if left uncontrolled could result to chronically high blood sugar levels, causing several symptoms and potentially leading to serious complications. Type 2 Diabetes in children is a growing problem. Endocrinology is the study of cell-to-cell signaling that occurs via specific chemicals (hormones) travelling through the bloodstream to influence remote targets. An endocrinologist is a specially trained clinician who is qualified for diagnosis of conditions that affect the endocrine glands and hormones. The following germane questions will be examined herein- What Is Type 2 Diabetes?, Causes and Symptoms, Prevention, Risk Factors and Treatment.

1.1 Symptoms

There is a chain reaction that can cause a variety of symptoms for Type 2 Diabetes which may be so mild not to notice at early stage.

The early symptoms may include:

- Fatigue
- Being very thirsty
- Peeing a lot

- Dry mouth
- Itchy skin
- Lack of energy
- Constant hunger
- Tingling or numbness in your hands or feet
- Blurry vision
- Being irritable

The latter symptoms, of which, having two or more requires medical attention, include:

- Slow-healing cuts or sores
- Dark patches on your skin
- Wounds that don't heal
- Neuropathy
- Yeast infections that keep coming back

1.2 What Causes Diabetes?

Insulin is the name of the hormone produced by the pancreas. This insulin is what enables the cells turn glucose from food into energy. It is a naturally occurring hormone. Type 2 Diabetes is exemplified by insulin resistance, wherein cells do not use insulin produced. This can damage cells in your pancreas. It could be as a result of cell dysfunction in the pancreas or with cell signaling and regulation, whereas for some people, the liver produces too much glucose. Combination of factors actually increases the risk of Type 2 Diabetes

The combination of things that can cause Type 2 Diabetes include:

> Extra weight.

> Broken beta cells

> Too much glucose from the liver

> Metabolic syndrome
> Bad communication between cells

1.3 Risk Factors For Type 2 Diabetes

Certain factors result in increased risk for Type 2 Diabetes, some of which are out of one's control, such as-

- Family- having blood relations who have Type 2 Diabetes.

- Age- risk is particularly high after age 45 though Type 2 Diabetes can develop at any age
- Ethnicity- It is proven that African-Americans, Latinos, Asian-Americans, and American Indians are at higher risk than Caucasians
- Health and medical history
  - Women who have a condition- polycystic ovarian syndrome
  - Being overweight which makes body cells more resistant to insulin.
  - Sedentary lifestyle
  - Having gestational diabetes while pregnant
  - Low HDL ("good") cholesterol
  - High blood pressure
  - Depression
  - Stress
  - Heart and blood vessel disease
  - Acanthosis nigricans, being a skin condition causing dark rashes around the neck or armpits
  - Smoking

1.4 The Risk Factors and Symptoms of Type 2 Diabetes In Children

Type 2 Diabetes in children is a growing phenomenon which a random blood sugar test may reveal. It is desirable to help lower a child's risk by encouraging the child to eat well and to be physically active every day. It is advised to see a Doctor immediately if a child has symptoms of diabetes since untreated diabetes can lead to serious and even life-threatening complications. Upon diagnosis with diabetes, the Doctor will need to determine if it is Type 1 or Type 2 before suggesting a specific treatment.

Risk factors for children include:

- sedentary lifestyle
- being overweight
- where mother is diagnosed of diabetes whilst pregnant with such child
- having a close family member with Type 2 Diabetes or birth weight of 9 pounds or more
- being American Indian, Alaska Native, African-American, Asian-American, Latino, or Pacific Islander

The notable symptoms of Type 2 Diabetes in children include:

- frequent infections
- increased urination

- sores that are slow to heal
- areas of darkened skin
- fatigue
- blurry vision

1.5 Diagnosis of Type 2 Diabetes

In dissecting this, some germane questions come to mind-What lifestyle changes can help me manage my diabetes? Is there a natural therapy that can cure diabetes ? Is There a Diabetes Cure? Are stem cells a possible cure for diabetes? What about islet cell transplantation or pancreas transplantation as a cure for diabetes?

Whereas it is proven that lifestyle changes can achieve remission in Type 2 Diabetes, in some cases despite the research on diabetes and advances in diabetes treatments, it cannot be said that there is a sure diabetes cure. Nonetheless, there are treatments, including simple things you can do daily, that are enormously beneficial.

Over time, it is proven that high blood sugar can damage and cause problems with the:

- Kidneys
- Heart and blood vessels
- Eyes
- Wound healing
- Nerves, which can lead to trouble with digestion
- Pregnancy

Routine screening for Type 2 Diabetes beginning at age 45, especially if overweight is highly recommended. Similarly, screening is also recommended for people who are under 45 and overweight if there are other heart disease or diabetes risk factors present.

Usually Doctors will conduct blood test on two different days to confirm, but where blood glucose is very high or you have a lot of symptoms, one test may be all you need. Thereafter, upon confirmation, you may need to see an endocrinologist who specializes in the treatment of diabetes.

Though Type 2 Diabetes can be effectively managed, it can affect virtually all your organs and lead to serious complications, including:

- ✓ skin problems, such as bacterial or fungal infections
- ✓ kidney damage and kidney failure
- ✓ Hypoglycemia
- ✓ nerve damage, or neuropathy
- ✓ poor circulation to the feet
- ✓ hearing impairment
- ✓ retinal damage, or retinopathy, and eye damage
- ✓ cardiovascular diseases such as high blood pressure, narrowing of the arteries, amongst others

Whereas, for diabetes complications during pregnancy, the following could be the downsides-

- ✓ increase your baby's risk of developing diabetes
- ✓ complicate labor
- ✓ harm baby's developing organs
- ✓ cause the baby to gain too much weight

Upon observing the symptoms of diabetes or prediabetes, you should see a doctor right away. Type 2 diabetes is usually diagnosed using the:

Glycated hemoglobin (A1C) Test: This blood test indicates sugar level for like an average of your blood glucose over the past 2 or 3 months. A hemoglobin A1C test is same as a glycosylated hemoglobin test. Whereas normal levels are below 5.7 percent, A1C level of 6.5 percent or higher on two separate tests means you have diabetes. During an oral glucose tolerance test, blood is drawn before and two hours after of taking a dose of glucose. If there is a confirmation of diabetes, the doctor will provide you with information about how to manage the disease, including:

- ✓ Dietary recommendations
- ✓ Ways to monitor blood glucose levels on your own
- ✓ Details of any medications that you need
- ✓ Physical activity recommendations

In addition to the A1C test, your Doctor will measure blood pressure, eye and foot examination and take blood and urine samples periodically to check cholesterol levels, thyroid function, liver function and kidney function.

Where A1C test is not available or hemoglobin variant - an uncommon form of hemoglobin, interferes with A1C test, the doctor may resort to use of the following tests to diagnose diabetes:

Fasting Plasma Glucose: A blood sample is taken after an overnight fast. It seeks to measure blood sugar on an empty stomach and you will not be able to eat or drink anything asides water for 8 hours before the test.

Oral Glucose Tolerance Test (OGTT): This checks the blood glucose before and 2 hours after taking a sweet drink to see how the body handles the sugar. Hence, it requires fasting overnight and then taking a sugary liquid at the doctor's office.

CHAPTER TWO

2.0 Fruit for a Diabetes Diet

Managing diabetes has to do with managing blood glucose, blood fats, blood pressure and weight, of which fruits and vegetables play a vital role. Diabetics, should eat some specified fruits as will be outlined. There are lots of benefits to eating fruit. Fruit is a great replacement for unhealthy processed sweets, such as pastries, cakes, and cookies, while providing disease-fighting antioxidants, and vitamins.

Generally speaking, the following is a list of common fruits:

- Tangerines
- Pineapple Grapefruit
- Banana
- Applesauce
- Blackberries
- Apples

- Avocado

- Apricots

- Blueberries

- Cantaloupe

- Dates

- Cherries

- Cranberries Figs

- Prunes

- Raisins

- Fruit cocktail

- Orange

- Pears

- Grapes

- Kiwi

- Papaya

- Peaches

- Mango

- Plums

- Raspberries

- Strawberries

- Watermelon

It is proven that fruits are loaded with vitamins, minerals and fiber just like vegetables, so you need to count it as part of your meal plan not only to satisfy your sweet tooth and get the extra nutrition you are looking for. Whereas, Dried fruit and 100% natural fruit juice are also nutritious, the portion sizes are small so they may not be as filling as other choices, the best choices, being, those that are fresh, frozen or canned without added sugars.

The fiber in whole fruits helps to keep blood sugar levels in check. Of the three main macronutrients in food — protein, fat, and carbohydrates, the last, directly affect blood sugar levels, and this includes the carbohydrates in fruit. People with Type 2 Diabetes must pay attention to their carbohydrate intake. It is proven that eating whole fruits — especially blueberries, grapes, and apples — significantly reduces the risk for Type 2 Diabetes. On the flip side, non natural fruit juices actually increase the risk for diabetes.

2.1 Tips for Diabetes Friendly Fruits

For a healthy diet, you need fruits due to the beneficial nutrients fruits provide just as you need vegetables and grains, however, with Type 2 Diabetes, it is equally important to keep track of the carbs.

Of note, antioxidants (common with fruits having a variety of bright colors and full flavors) are important in a diabetes diet because they help reduce inflammation caused by oxidative stress, which contribute to complications of diabetes.

Including more fiber (common in fruits like apples, pears, and peaches) in diet means better blood sugar. Fiber is especially important for a diabetes diet because it is not digestible, so it raises blood sugar.

2.2 Counting Fruit Carbs

Since there is no one specific amount of carbohydrate intake for all people with diabetes, it is important to count your carbs(spread them out throughout the day) and work with your healthcare providers to come up with a suitable target in balancing fruit with proteins and other sources of healthy carbohydrates.

2.3 Tips For Carbohydrate Counters

Fruit can be eaten in exchange for other sources of carbohydrate in meal such as starches, grains, or dairy. Hence, it is important to note the grams of carbohydrate of servings for whole fruit or frozen or canned fruit, berries, melons and fruit juice for restraint in portion sizes. It is trite that having a small piece of whole fruit or a ½ cup of fruit salad for dessert is a great complement to the non-starchy vegetables, small portion of starch and protein foods .

2.4 Tips For Using the Glycemic Index

Fruit is encouraged when using the Glycemic Index to guide food choices because majority of fruits have low Glycemic Index (GI) because of their fructose and fiber, though Melons, dried fruits such as dates, raisins, likewise and pineapple have medium Glycemic Index (GI) values.

2.5 Choosing the Best Fruits to Eat for Diabetes

Fruit is not off-limits for type 2 diabetes because fruit is a good alternative to sugar-laden desserts since it can satisfy your sweet tooth while delivering fiber, antioxidants, amongst others. Some colorful, flavorful fruits of all varieties can be beneficial in a diabetes diet; nonetheless, count the carbs and eat fruit in moderation. Choose whole fruits instead of fruit juices. When in doubt, then endeavour to consult the glycemic load, a scale that helps to measure how much a serving of a certain food is likely to spike blood sugar, to pick a diabetes-friendly fruit.

Best options:

These high-antioxidant fruits should be considered as best options to eat for a healthy diabetes diet:

- Grapes

- Apples

- Berries

- Citrus fruits

- Papaya

- Cantaloupe

- Pineapple

- Mango

- Apricots

Options To Be Weary of

Of note, fruits and vegetables lower the risk of developing many health conditions including high blood pressure, heart diseases, strokes, obesity and certain cancers. But everyone responds to food differently. Testing blood sugars before and after eating fruit can help determine which fruits are best. The context in which fruit is taken is likewise of importance, hence, pair your fruit with protein and note that the riper a fruit is, the higher its Glycemic Index, which means it will raise your blood sugar more than a food with a low Glycemic Index.

Remarkably, it is important for diabetics to regulate their blood sugar levels at all times. Whilst there is no such thing as a "bad" fruit, if you have diabetes, there is need to take caution with some fruits since all the different kinds of fruits in nature's basket have different effects on blood sugar level, which is measured by the Glycaemic Index. Because fruit is a carbohydrate, it will affect your blood sugar and you cannot have unlimited amounts of just any fruit. Hence, fruits that are absorbed quickly and aiding in having quick burst of energy are categorised as high-glycaemic index foods, whereas fruits that are digested slower with more sustained energy release, are categorised as low-GI foods.

Fruits with a low Glycaemic Index are always the recommended safe choice for diabetics; examples of low-GI fruit are apples, pears, oranges, peaches, plums and strawberries. Medium to high-GI fruits (such as banana, pineapple, watermelon, sweet melon and papaya), can be taken by diabetics only if taken after exercising for at least one hour to avoid a high sugar spike. Overall, striking a balance is important. A dietician can teach you how this can be done in a safe and sensible manner. The bad options are -

- Canned fruit in syrup

- Dried fruit: Especially varieties that have been coated in yogurt, chocolate or sugar; these contain a large amount of carbohydrates for a small portion. Two tablespoons of raisins has the same amount of carbohydrate as one cup of raspberries or one small piece of fruit. Replace dried fruit with fresh fruit to add volume to your meal plan and reduce the sugar content.

- Packaged juices: Fruit juices can be high in natural sugars and because they have less fibre than the whole fruits, they are not as beneficial.

  Because you can get through a lot of juice within a relatively short period of time, compared to eating the actual fruit, you may end up loading up with a lot of carbs over that period. Depending on how your diabetes is managed, this can result in your blood glucose levels going up, and may affect your weight in the long term as well.

  That is why you are better off eating the actual fruit and avoiding juices. If you want to drink fruit juice, then my advice would be to limit it to a maximum of a small glass, once a day; limit it to a maximum of 1 small glass a day because drinking more than that will only increase your blood glucose levels and make you gain weight.

Many people tend to have juice with their meals, but my advice would be if you have it with your meal then look at how to reduce the carbohydrate. So, for example, if you usually have a couple of slices of bread with your breakfast, on the day that you decide to have a small glass of juice with your breakfast, you may be better off sacrificing one slice of bread to make room for the extra carbs from the juice. I'm not saying do this every day, but that is an option to ensure that you do not have to deal with high blood glucose levels as a result of the juice.

- Fresh juices that are part of fad cleanses: Unless you are experiencing hypoglycemia, non natural fruit juice should be avoided. Think about how many oranges it takes to make one cup of juice - many more than one. One eight ounce cup of orange juice contains 30 grams of carbohydrate, 30 grams of sugar and no fiber.

The body doesn't have to do a great deal of work to break down the sugar in juice, therefore it is metabolized quickly and raises blood sugar within minutes. Juice can also tack on extra calories without affecting your satiety and therefore can prevent weight loss and even promote weight gain. Swap fruit juice for whole fruit, and limit your portions to no more than two-to-three per day.

The not so advisable fruit either because they have a higher glycemic index or because most people overeat them are-

a. Cherries: Most people don't stop eating cherries at just a handful, which is why eating cherries will usually result in blood sugar spikes. Similar to grapes, one cherry contains one gram of carbohydrate. If you find that yourself snacking on a big bowl of cherries, it's probably best to avoid them altogether.

b. Pineapple: Fresh pineapple is delicious and sweet, especially when it's very ripe, which makes it a high Glycemic Index food. Depending on how you slice it, the thickness and width can change the amount of carbohydrates and make it easy to overeat.

If you must eat pineapple, stick to a 1/2 cup serving and aim to eat it with a meal or a protein-rich food such as low-fat Greek yogurt or low-fat cottage cheese. Avoid canned pineapple that has been sweetened with sugar. If you are buying canned pineapple, purchase the no sugar added variety.

c. Apples: Apples, also rich in polyphenols, offer something extra-special: a pre-set serving size. Be sure to eat the skin, where much of fiber is found. Fiber is helpful because it fills you up and it can slow the absorption of sugar in the blood.

2.6 The Basic Five-A-Day Plan

In having that perfect habit of a healthy diet for diabetics, then it is desireable to consider a portion of fruit and veg, which is roughly what can fit in the palm. Of note, try to spread your intake through the day rather than having all in one go. A good example is-

- a handful of grapes

- 3 tablespoon of vegetables

- 1 tablespoon of dried fruits

- a medium size apple, pear or banana

- a bowl of salad

Serving For Breakfast:

You can simply opt for fruit salad topped with no added sugar yoghurt and choose low-fat yogurt if you are managing your weight.

Also you can add sliced banana to your cereal for breakfast. Remember to reduce your usual amount of cereal to make room for fruit. Equally, try adding mushrooms and tomatoes with your cooked breakfast.

Serving For Lunch:

Try having a healthy side salad with sandwich. Replace snacks with fruits and veg e.g. fruit salads, raw vegetables or vegetable sticks.

Serving For Supper:

For evening meals dish out the vegetables first like carrots, aubergines, broccoli, cabbages etc. and let that form the biggest part of the plate and add more vegetables to your casseroles, stews, soups etc.

2.7 Useful Tips On Fruit And Vegetables

Fruit and vegetables have different mix of nutrients, so, challenge yourself to try different fruit or veg whenever possible. They are better eaten raw as some nutrients are lost through cooking. It is important to have a range of fruits and veg to get more goodness. If you prefer them cooked, try steaming, poaching or microwaving rather than boiling in a lot of water; then, add some spices. Nonetheless, be careful with dried fruits, fruit juices and smoothies

As for fruit in tins, choose the one that is tinned in the natural juice rather than syrup; then, always read the label.

CHAPTER THREE

3.0 Food for a Diabetes Diet

Foods that are nutritious and have low Glycemic Index (GI) are helpful in managing blood glucose levels. Besides nutrient content, the Glycemic Index (GI) of a food may also help in making healthy choices. Understanding how different foods affect blood sugar is important to follow a healthy diet for diabetes. For instance, protein and fats do not directly impact blood sugar, nonetheless, they are to be consumed in moderation to reduce calories. On the other hand, carbohydrates, which are found to the largest degree in grains, bread, fruit, milk, sweets and starchy vegetables, are broken down into glucose in the blood faster than other types of food, thereby raising blood sugar. Hence, it is important to monitor portions for foods with a high carbohydrate content. Working with a certified diabetes educator or a registered dietitian to determine personalized daily suitable carbohydrate goal is desirable and to help formulate a helpful guideline.

Lower glycemic index (GI) foods area better choice for people with diabetes. Diabetics can enjoy a wide range of foods and in some cases, such can even help reverse Type 2 Diabetes. Following through a super Type 2 Diabetes diet is a balancing act that requires having a variety of healthy carbohydrates, fats, and proteins. The secret is choosing the right combination of foods that will help keep your blood sugar level and avoid food that will fuel the symptoms of diabetes ranging from the frequent urination, fatigue, dizziness, headaches, and mood changes of low blood sugar.

Thus, in choosing the most diabetes-friendly food, it should be noted that sugar, soda, candy, and other packaged or processed snacks and processed carbohydrates should be limited. The other things to be noted in choosing the most diabetes-friendly foods from each food class are:

3.1 What Foods High in Protein Are Beneficial for Type 2 Diabetes Patients?

In addition to getting enough fiber, having protein-rich foods can help keep you satiated and promote weight loss, thereby reducing insulin resistance, the hallmark of diabetes.

Lean protein, low in saturated fat, is good for people with diabetes. For those on a vegan or vegetarian diet, getting sufficient and right balance of protein may be more challenging, but they can rely on foods like beans and nuts to get your fix. However, processed or packaged foods should be avoided or limited in diabetes diet because, in addition to added sugars and processed carbohydrates, these foods are often high in sodium and therefore may increase blood pressure, resulting in the risk of heart disease or stroke, being the two common complications of diabetes. It is important to keep blood pressure in check when managing diabetes, hence, the best options remains:

- Skinless turkey

- Canned tuna in water

- Plain, nonfat Greek yogurt

- Skinless chicken

- Fatty fish, like sockeye salmon

- Beans and legumes

- Eggs

- Raw, unsalted nuts, like walnuts (in moderation)

Flowing from the above, the worst options are:

- Hot dogs

- Sausages and pepperoni

- Deli meats, like bologna, ham, roast beef, and turkey

- Beef jerky

- Sweetened or flavored nuts, like honey-roasted or spicy

- Sweetened protein shakes or smoothies

- Bacon

3.2 What Are the Best Grains Beneficial for Type 2 Diabetes Patients?

Any type of grain contains carbs, so counting carbs and practicing portion control are keys to keep your blood sugar level steady. Whereas, grains in the form of popular foods such as white bread, as well as sugary, processed, or packaged grains, should be avoided or limited to avoid unwanted blood sugar spikes, vitamin-rich whole grains in a healthy diabetes diet is good, hence, contrary to popular belief, not all carbs are off-limits for persons managing diabetes. On the other hand, refined white flour doesn't contain the same vitamins, minerals, fiber, and health benefits as whole grains. These Vitamin-rich whole grains contain fiber that is beneficial for digestive health. In fact, fiber can also promote feelings of fullness, preventing you from reaching for unhealthy snacks, and it can help slow the rise of blood sugar. Plus, whole grains contain healthy vitamins, minerals, and phytochemicals that are healthy for anyone.

Just keep in mind that the following are desirable options (to be taken in moderation):

- Whole-grain breads, such as 100 percent whole-wheat bread

- Whole-grain cereal, such as steel-cut oats

- Whole-wheat pasta

- Wild or brown rice

Also keep in mind that the following are worst options:

- Sugary breakfast cereals

- White pasta

- White rice

- Pastries

- White bread

3.3 What Are the Best Types of Dairy For People With Diabetes?

It is always good to settle for fat-free dairy options to keep calories down and unhealthy saturated fats at bay. When picked well and eaten in moderation, dairy products can be a great choice for people with diabetes. However, keep fat content in mind, as being overweight or obese can reduce insulin sensitivity, causing prediabetes to progress to full-blown diabetes.

Whenever possible, the best options to consider are:

- Nonfat, low-sodium cottage cheese

- Skim milk

- Reduced-fat cheese (to be taken in moderation)

- Nonfat plain Greek yogurt

- Nonfat, unsweetened kefir

The following options are not advisable:

- Full-fat, sweetened kefir

- Full-fat or reduced-fat cottage cheese

- Full-fat yogurt

- Full-fat cheese

- Full-fat or reduced-fat (2 percent) milk, especially chocolate and flavored milks

3.4 What Are the Best Types of Vegetables for People With Diabetes?

Vegetables are an important food group to include in any healthy diet since they are full of fiber and nutrients. No starchy varieties are low in carbohydrates, hence, good for people with diabetes as it aids to gain control over blood sugar level. Frozen vegetables without sauce are as nutritious as fresh, and even low-sodium canned veggies is a good choice. Be sure to watch your sodium intake to avoid high blood pressure, and consider draining and rinsing salted canned vegetables before eating; try choosing low-sodium or sodium-free canned vegetables.

However the general rule is: Try filling half your plate with nonstarchy veggies. Whenever you crave for mashed white potatoes, try mashed cauliflower. Better still, try out sweet potatoes, which people with diabetes can enjoy safely in moderation.

Best nonstarchy veggie options:

- Cruciferous veggies, like broccoli

- Artichoke hearts

- Asparagus

- Brussels sprouts

- Greens, like spinach, kale, and Swiss chard

- Peppers

- Cucumbers

- Onions

Veggies to enjoy in moderation:

- Corn

- White potatoes

- Sweet potatoes

- Beets

- Yams

- Peas

3.5 What Are the Best Types of Fat And Bad Fat For Diabetes?

Whereas, the right fat, such as monounsaturated fats found in avocados, and almonds or the polyunsaturated fats found in walnuts and sunflower oil, can help curb unhealthy cravings, lose weight, and attain better control over blood sugar, saturated fats can harm the heart. Succinctly, it is important to distinguish good fat from bad fat.

Best options are identified hereunder:

- Nut butters

- Nuts, like almonds, and walnuts

- Plant-based oils, like soybean oil, olive oil, and sunflower oil

- Seeds, like flaxseed and chia seed

- Edamame

- Avocados

- Fish, like salmon and tuna

- Olives

Worst options are identified hereunder:

- Fast food

- Full-fat dairy products

- Processed sweets, like doughnuts, cakes, and cookies

- Beef, veal, lamb, and pork

- Coconut and palm oil

- Packaged snacks, like crackers, corn chips, and potato chips

3.6 What Are The Best 10 Superfood That Are Especially Good For Those With Diabetes?

1. **Non-starchy vegetables**: This category of vegetables go a long way in satisfying boosting intake of vitamins, minerals, fiber, and phytochemicals. The Non-starchy vegetables are low in calories and carbohydrates, making them some of the few foods that people with diabetes can relish. It is proven that people given a low-calorie diet consisting of non-starchy vegetables might successfully reverse type 2 diabetes. The Non-starchy vegetables have fewer carbs per serving. They include everything from artichokes and asparagus to broccoli and beets.

2. **Unsweetened Greek yogurt**: With a low GI score, unsweetened Greek yogurt is full of healthy probiotics, calcium, and protein and studies have shown a 14 percent lower risk of type 2 diabetes with daily yogurt consumption. It is nutritious to t top unsweetened Greek yogurt with nuts and low GI fruits such as blackberries, blueberries, or raspberries. Unsweetened Greek yogurt is a better option than regular yogurt due to its higher protein and lower carbohydrate content. Hence, it is

important to check nutrition labels, as some brands have a higher carbohydrate content than others, due to additions such as syrup flavorings, sweeteners, toppers, or fruit preserves.

3. **Tomatoes**: Tomatoes like other non-starchy fruits, have a low GI ranking, as such, whether eaten raw or cooked, tomatoes are full of lycopene, a powerful substance that may reduce the risk of cancer (especially prostate cancer), heart disease, and macular degeneration.

Tomato consumption might help reduce cardiovascular risk that's associated with type 2 diabetes. It is proven that 200 grams of raw tomato (or about 1.5 medium tomatoes) each day reduced blood pressure in people with type 2 diabetes.

4. **Blueberries and other berries**: They have some of the highest antioxidant levels of any fruit or vegetable and may reduce the risk of heart disease and cancer and have anti-inflammatory properties. From vision-protecting vitamin C to filling fiber, blueberries are proven antioxidant powerhouses.

Strawberries, raspberries, and blackberries are equally good choices for people with diabetes.

5. **Oranges and other citrus**: The pulpiness of oranges and grapefruit provide a great source of fiber which can be maximized by eating the whole fruit rather than drinking just the juice since it is proven that eating citrus fruits could lower the risk of diabetes in women, but drinking the fruit juice could increase that risk. The citrus with the lowest GI score is grapefruit which has one of the lowest GI scores of all fruits.

Whereas the average orange has a GI score of 40 while unsweetened orange juice has a GI score of 50.

6. **Wild salmon and other fish with omega-3 fatty acids**: Wild salmon is full of vitamin D and selenium for healthy hair, skin, nails, and bones and it is equally loaded with omega-3 fatty acids, which may lower risk of heart disease. In addition, other nutrient-dense fish include herring, sardines, and mackerel. Fish oil is another source of omega-3 fatty acids. Fish and other protein foods do not contain

carbs, hence, do not increase blood sugar levels. Adding salmon to a meal can help slow digestion of other foods eaten at that meal.

7. **Walnuts, flax seeds, and other nuts and seeds**: It is proven that people who eat nuts regularly have less risk of developing diabetes. Nuts generally have very low GI scores as such, substituting nuts and other healthy fats for carbs can help lower blood sugar. Whilst a good number of nuts provide healthy fats and can curb hunger, two powerful ones are walnuts and flax seeds which contain magnesium, fiber, and omega-3 fatty acids. Walnuts contain alpha-linolenic acid, an essential fatty acid that boosts heart health and lowers cholesterol and are full of vitamin E, folic acid, zinc, and protein.

8. **Beans**: Beans is high in fiber and protein, making them a great option for vegetarians and vegans. It is among nature's most nutritious foods because it delivers essential minerals like magnesium and potassium. It is proven that beans is a good way to

control glycemic levels in people with type 2 diabetes and can also reduce the risk of coronary heart disease.

9. **Kale and other leafy green vegetables**: Kale is the king of super healthy greens that contains chemicals called glucosinolates that help neutralize cancer-causing substances. Kale is full of potassium and has been shown to help manage blood pressure.

Kale provides more than 100 percent of the recommended daily intake of vitamin A and K. On the other hand, collard greens are another leafy green that packs a ton of nutrients into a small package.

10. **Barley, lentils, and other whole grains**: The grain keeps blood sugar levels stable. Equally, lentils are another good option since they provide B vitamins, iron, complex carbohydrates, and protein. Eating whole grains helps decrease the risk of developing type 2 diabetes, if the right type is taken. Whole grains are full of antioxidants and soluble and insoluble fiber that are beneficial to metabolize fats and keep the digestive track healthy. It is proven that

people who regularly eat hulled barley typically have lower blood cholesterol.

CHAPTER FOUR

4.0 Lifestyle Changes That Can Help Manage Diabetes

Upon being diagnosed with diabetes, there is a lot you can do to improve your health. Of note, Type 2 diabetes is on the rise around the world. Diabetes can be treated and controlled, hence, the best way to avoid the complications of diabetes is to manage the diabetes well by sticking with Diabetes medications, eating food good for diabetes, shedding pounds, exercising regularly, maintaining a healthy weight, regularly checking blood glucose, whilst not downplaying seeing the doctor regularly to check for early warning signs.

In view of the fact that diabetes increases the risk of cardiovascular disease, your Doctor will also monitor your blood pressure and blood cholesterol levels. Hence, managing type 2 diabetes requires working closely with your doctor, but a lot of the results depend on your commitment. It may also be helpful to bring your family into the loop so that they can help in an emergency. Following your diabetes treatment plan takes round-the-clock commitment; learn more about how to live better every day. These management strategies can have a dramatic impact on blood sugar levels and the progression of Type 2 Diabetes and are proven ways to take an active role in diabetes care and enjoy a healthier future.

4.1 Lose Weight Especially Belly Fat To Help Lower Glucose Levels

Eating healthy foods are simple ways to start taking weight off. Losing just 5 to 10 percent of body weight can make a difference since shedding pounds can improve blood sugar levels and help keep Type 2 Diabetes under control. Shedding weight equally helps to prevent prediabetes from progressing to full-blown Type 2 Diabetes and help halts the advancement of Type 2 Diabetes. A healthy diet and regular aerobic exercise will reduce weight in the stomach area. Abdominal fat tends to increase insulin since people who carry most of their fat in their belly (referred to as having an apple-shaped body) are more prone to Type 2 Diabetes than those with fat mostly in the thighs, hips, and buttocks (referred to as having a pear-shaped body).

4.2 Stick To Your Diabetes Eating Plan

Have healthy snacks with you regularly to reduce the likelihood to snack on empty calories. A registered dietitian can teach you how to monitor your carbohydrate intake and let you know about how many carbohydrates you need to eat with your meals and snacks to keep your blood sugar levels stable. Try to center your diet around:

- Fewer calories

- Fewer refined carbohydrates

- Fewer foods containing saturated fats

- More foods with fiber

- More vegetables and fruits

4.3 Exercise Regularly And Have Eye Examination

Exercise helps keep you fit, so, endeavour to choose activities you enjoy, such as walking, swimming, regular weightlifting and biking, so that you can make them part of your daily routine. Also, try to schedule yearly physical and routine eye exams wherein the Doctor will ask about your nutrition and activity level and look for any diabetes-related complications. An eye care specialist will normally check signs of retinal damage and cataracts.

More so, ensure to reduce the amount of time you spend in inactive activities, such as watching Television. You can help keep Type 2 Diabetes under control with daily exercise sessions since when you engage in physical activity, such as walking, your muscle contractions push glucose out of your blood into your cells.

4.4 Monitor Blood Sugar and Control Sleep Apnea

Careful monitoring of blood sugar is the best means of ensuring that your blood sugar level remains within your target range. Of note, overweight people with Type 2 Diabetes also have sleep apnea, which is a condition in which a person stops breathing temporarily while sleeping, and such people are at higher risk of death from diabetes complications such as heart attack and stroke. Severe cases of sleep apnea may need to be treated with surgery but less severe cases can be managed by losing weight.

4.5 Stress Management

It becomes easier to observe diabetes care routine if you manage your stress. Don't forget to get plenty of sleep. Moreso, poorly managed stress can make blood sugar levels harder to control. So, employ top-notch stress busters for diabetes such as: yoga, meditation, prioritizing your tasks, massage, and soothing music, and try using relaxation techniques to chase away stress.

4.6 If You Can Not Stay Away From Alcohol, Drink With Moderation

If you choose to drink, do so responsibly since alcohol can cause high or low blood sugar. Only drink with a meal or snack, and do not forget to include the calories from any alcohol intake to your daily calorie count.

4.7 Keep Up With Your Medical Appointments

Those in this category are your doctor, diabetes educator, ophthalmologist, dentist, podiatrist, and other health care professionals.

4.8 Avoid Smoking

Consider ways to help you stop smoking or using other types of tobacco. The effects of smoking for diabetics is massive since it increases the risk of various diabetes complications, including:

- Heart disease

- Kidney disease

- Eye disease

- Stroke

- Reduced blood flow in the legs and feet

- Nerve damage

- Premature death

4.9 Be Committed To Keeping Your Blood Pressure And Cholesterol Under Control

High blood pressure can damage your blood vessels and is harmful like diabetes, hence, both can lead to a heart attack, stroke or other life-threatening conditions. High cholesterol is equally harmful. Thus, reduced-fat diet and exercising regularly is recommended.

4.10 Be Committed To Managing Your Diabetes

You have to learn all you can about diabetes working with your Doctor or primary care provider, diabetes nurse educator, and dietitian to know how best to manage your condition. Then ensure to follow your Doctor's instructions for managing your blood sugar level.

4.11 Have The Necessary Recommended Vaccine

The likelihood of having other illness is high for diabetics, hence the following vaccines are helpful:

- Flu vaccine

- Hepatitis B vaccine

- Pneumonia vaccine

4.12 Pay Attention to Your Teeth

The likelihood of having gum infections is high for diabetics, so it is advisable to pay attention to your overall dental health by brushing your teeth at least twice a day with fluoride toothpaste and floss your teeth once a day. See your dentist if your gums bleed or look red or swollen.

4.13 Take Care of Your Feet

Since high blood sugar reduce blood flow and damage the nerves in your feet, the resultant cuts and blisters can lead to serious infections. This can cause pain, tingling or loss of sensation in your feet. So it is recommended that-

- Don't go barefoot, indoors or outdoors.

- Moisturize your feet and ankles with lotion

- Wash your feet daily in lukewarm water.

- Check your feet daily for calluses, blisters, sores, foot ulcer, an open etc. Consult your doctor if you notice any of these.

- Dry your feet gently, especially between the toes.

4.14 Consider Having A Daily Aspirin

Your Doctor may recommend taking a low dose of aspirin every day to help reduce your risk of heart attack and stroke if you have diabetes and other cardiovascular risk factors. Where there is no additional cardiovascular risk factor, the risk of bleeding from aspirin use likely outweighs any benefits of aspirin use.

No doubt, careful management of Type 2 Diabetes can reduce your risk of serious even life-threatening complications. These tips as deduced from the foregoing exposition are helpful:

1. Do not shy away from admitting that you have Type 2 Diabetes and ask your diabetes treatment team for help when you need it.

2. Have regular diabetes checkups . Schedule a yearly physical exam and regular eye exams; observe regular physicals or routine eye exams.

3. Eat right by making healthy eating and physical activity part of your daily routine

4. Since High blood sugar can weaken your immune system ensure to keep your vaccinations up to date. Get a flu shot every year.

5. Since Diabetes may leave you prone to more-serious gum infections, endeavour to take care of your teeth; brush and floss your teeth regularly and schedule recommended dental exams. If your gums bleed or look red or swollen, consult your dentist.

6. Do not neglect caring for your feet by washing your feet daily in lukewarm water, drying them gently(especially between the toes) and moisturize them with lotion. Consult your Doctor if you have a sore blisters, cuts, sores, redness

and swelling or other foot problem that is not healing.

7. Eating healthy food and exercising regularly is desireable to keep your blood pressure and cholesterol under control since it can go a long way in controlling high blood pressure and cholesterol.

8. Do note that smoking increases your risk of various diabetes complications so if you smoke or use other types of tobacco, ask your Doctor to help you quit.

9. Do note that Alcohol, as well as drink mixers, can cause either high or low blood sugar, depending on how much you drink and if you eat at the same time, so, if you drink alcohol, do so responsibly. If you choose to drink, do so in moderation and always with a meal.

CHAPTER FIVE

5.0 Medication And Treatment for Type 2 Diabetes

A Doctor might combine drugs from different classes to help control blood sugar in several different ways since the decision about which medications are best depends on many factors such as blood sugar level and other health problems. Of note, each of these medications can cause side effects and it may take some time to find the best medication or combination of medications suitable for individuals. A hemoglobin A1C test can provide more information about average blood sugar. If blood pressure or cholesterol levels are a problem, you may need medications to address those needs. If your body can not produce sufficient insulin, you may need insulin therapy.

Of note, some people who have Type 2 Diabetes can achieve their target blood sugar levels with diet and exercise alone. However, some require diabetes medications or insulin therapy.

5.1 Medications For Type 2 Diabetes

You can effectively manage Type 2 Diabetes as will be discovered upon an examination of examples of possible treatments for Type 2 Diabetes. Type 2 diabetes treatment is never a one size fits all, so your Doctor will tell you how often you should check your blood glucose levels since the goal is to stay within a specific range. In some cases, lifestyle changes are enough to keep Type 2 Diabetes under control whereas in other cases, there are several medications that may help.

Thus, Diabetes treatment recommendations tend to vary from person to person; there are many drug options available, and the initial approach might need to be changed as treatment progresses. When lifestyle changes alone can't control blood sugar, your Doctor may prescribe medicine. Each of these medications can cause side effects and it may take some time to find the best medication or combination of medications to treat your diabetes.

Where blood pressure or cholesterol levels are a problem, you may need medications to address those needs as well.

A hemoglobin A1C test can provide more information about average blood sugar. If your body can not make enough insulin, you may need insulin therapy. Amylin analogs can also aid weight loss and requires an additional shot with each meal. In addition to diabetes medications, your doctor might prescribe low-dose aspirin therapy as well as blood pressure and cholesterol-lowering medications.

There are several medications that may help. Some of these medications are:

- **Meglitinides or Glinides**: These are fast-acting, short-duration medications that stimulate your pancreas to release more insulin. They are fast-acting, short-duration medications that stimulate your pancreas to release more insulin. It triggers beta cells in the pancreas to release insulin, are taken before each meal. These medications — such as repaglinide (Prandin) and nateglinide (Starlix) — work like sulfonylureas by stimulating the pancreas to secrete more insulin, but they are faster acting, and the duration of their effect in the body is shorter. They also have a risk of causing low blood sugar and weight gain.

- **Sulfonylureas:** This helps the body produce more insulin and it triggers insulin-releasing beta cells in your pancreas; usually taken one or two times a day, before meals. Examples include glyburide, glimepiride, chlorpropamide, and tolazamide. Possible side effects include low blood sugar and weight gain

- **Metformin (Glucophage, Glumetza, others)**: It can lower your blood sugar levels and improve how your body responds to insulin. Of note, it is the first medication prescribed for type 2 diabetes because it works by lowering glucose production in the liver and improving your body's sensitivity to insulin so that your body uses insulin more effectively. Other oral medications may be added to drug therapy with metformin if metformin and lifestyles changes aren't enough to control your blood sugar level. Nausea and diarrhea are possible side effects of metformin.

- **Glucagon-like Peptide-1 Receptor Agonists**: This helps slow digestion and improve blood sugar levels

- **Sodium-Glucose Cotransporter-2 Inhibitors**: This helps help prevent the kidneys from reabsorbing sugar into the blood and sending it out in your urine. They slow the kidney's reabsorption of glucose, allow more blood sugar to leave your body via urine and these drugs prevent the kidneys from reabsorbing sugar into the blood. Instead, the sugar is excreted in the urine. Examples include canagliflozin (Invokana), dapagliflozin (Farxiga) and empagliflozin (Jardiance).

- **Dipeptidyl Peptidase-4 Inhibitors:** This is a milder medication that helps reduce blood sugar levels. They help reduce blood sugar levels, but tend to have a very modest effect. They stop the normal breakdown rate of a compound called GLP-1, help lower the blood sugar level. Examples of these medications are sitagliptin (Januvia), saxagliptin (Onglyza) and linagliptin (Tradjenta). They do not cause weight gain though may cause joint pain and increase your risk of pancreatitis.

- **GLP-1 receptor agonists:** They help promote weight loss and can be taken daily or weekly. These injectable medications slow digestion and help lower blood sugar levels. Their use is often associated with weight loss. Exenatide (Byetta, Bydureon), liraglutide (Victoza) and semaglutide (Ozempic) are examples of GLP-1 receptor agonists. Possible side effects include nausea and an increased risk of pancreatitis.

- **Thiazolidinediones:** This helps make the body more sensitive to insulin. Like metformin, these medications — including rosiglitazone (Avandia) and pioglitazone (Actos) — make the body's tissues more sensitive to insulin; it improves the way your body uses insulin, may also lower blood sugar production in the liver. Pioglitazone is an example. It makes your body more sensitive to insulin. However, they have been linked to weight gain and other more-serious side effects, such as an increased risk of heart failure and anemia, hence, these medications generally are not first-choice treatments.

5.2 Tips for Navigating a Type 2 Diabetes Treatment Plan

Side effects of diabetes medications may include gastrointestinal illnesses, dizziness, or fatigue and a side effect of metformin may be weight loss, while using insulin injections may contribute to weight gain. So, if treating diabetes involves oral or injectable medication, make sure you understand the side effects of everything you take. Equally, if you have questions on your current treatment or feel it needs to be adjusted, talk to your Doctor. Then, confirm whether your medication regimen could lead to low blood sugar.

Cholesterol-lowering medications, aspirin and some blood pressure drugs can't be used during pregnancy, as such, women with type 2 diabetes may need to alter their treatment during pregnancy. Thus, many women may require insulin therapy during pregnancy.

5.3 What You Can Do When In Doubt

If your blood sugar is consistently out of your target range, or if you are not sure what to do in a certain situation, contact your Doctor or diabetes educator.

5.3.1 Preparing For Appointment For A Type 2 Diabetes Diagnosis

Whenever you can, it's a good idea to prepare for appointments with your health care team.

Your health care team will probably diagnose your Type 2 Diabetes and may continue to treat your diabetes or may refer you to a Doctor who specializes in hormonal disorders (endocrinologist). If your blood sugar levels are very high, your Doctor may send you to the hospital for treatment. Your health care team also may include these specialists:

- Dietitian

- Certified diabetes educator

- Foot doctor (podiatrist)

- Doctor who specializes in eye care (ophthalmologist)

5.3.2 What You Can Do Upon Making An Appointment With A Doctor

Having writing materials, either a notebook or your computer or tablet can help keep track of important information on your diabetes. Write down symptoms, including any that may seem unrelated to diabetes.

Be aware of any pre-appointment restrictions. You may need to avoid eating or drinking anything but water for eight hours for a fasting glucose test or for four hours for a pre-meal test; simply ensure that when making an appointment, ask if you should fast or not.

5.3.3 Helpful Questions To Ask Your Doctor

Hereunder set out are some information to help you get ready for your appointment and know what to expect from your Doctor. For Type 2 Diabetes, the questions set out below can help you make the most of your time with your Doctor:

- ✓ How much exercise should I get each day?

- ✓ Do I need to take medicine or insulin shots? How often?

- ✓ How often do I need to monitor my blood sugar, and what is my target range?

- ✓ What changes in my diet would help me manage my blood sugar?

- ✓ How will I know if I'm managing my diabetes well?

- ✓ How often do I need to be monitored for diabetes complications? What specialists do I need to see?

- ✓ Should I see a dietitian to help with meal planning?

- ✓ Do I need to take the medicine at a particular time of the day?

- ✓ I have other medical problems. How can I best manage these conditions together?

- ✓ Are there resources available if I am having trouble paying for diabetes supplies?

- ✓ Are there brochures or other printed material that I can take with me? What websites do you recommend?

5.3.4 Likely Questions To Expect From Your Doctor

Your doctor is likely to ask you a number of questions, including:

✓ Do you sit for long periods of time?

✓ What's a typical day's diet like?

✓ Do you understand your treatment plan and feel confident you can follow it?

✓ How are you coping with diabetes?

✓ Do you know what to do if your blood sugar is too low or too high?

✓ What challenges are you experiencing in managing your diabetes?

✓ Have you experienced any low blood sugar?

✓ Are you exercising and what type of exercise? How often?

5.4 Is There A Natural Therapy That Can Cure Diabetes?

Some natural supplements have been proven to help improve diabetes. However, endeavour to always check with your Doctor before taking any of these natural supplement. Emotional stress affects blood sugar levels, hence, learning to relax is important in managing diabetes. Some natural therapies such as deep abdominal breathing, progressive muscle relaxation, guided imagery, and biofeedback can help relieve stress.

Of note, supplements don't cure diabetes either. Whereas some natural supplements may interact dangerously with your diabetes medication, while others may not.

5.5 Are Stem Cells A Possible Cure For Diabetes?

Stem cells are cells that can develop into other types of cells. Scientists have had some success with stem cells precisely for Type 1 Diabetes. Stem cells definitely have prospects but cannot be said to be a treatment now.

5.6 Islet Cell Transplantation As A Cure For Diabetes

Islet cells sense blood sugar levels and make insulin. This cell come from a donor and is an evolving technology. A successful islet cell transplant can improve the quality of life for a person with diabetes since it provides more flexibility with meal planning and help protect against serious long-term diabetes complications such as heart disease, stroke, kidney disease, nerve and eye damage. Once transplanted successfully, the donor cells begin to make and release insulin in response to blood sugar levels, but the person receiving the transplant must take medicine for the rest of their life to prevent their body from rejecting the donor's cells.

5.7 Pancreas Transplantation As A Cure For Diabetes

A pancreatic transplant helps restore blood sugar control and it is done for those who also have end-stage disease. Getting a transplanted pancreas is a possibility for some people with Type 1 Diabetes. Just like any other patient having undergone transplant, the patient would need to take medicine for the rest of their life to help their body accept their new pancreas.

5.8 Complications That Affect Blood Sugar

Some notable complications for diabetics that may arise requiring immediate care due to the fact that the blood sugar is involved are hereunder set out:

5.8.1 Hyperglycemic Hyperosmolar Nonketotic Syndrome (HHNS): It is a life-threatening condition that can cause dry mouth, extreme thirst, drowsiness, confusion, dark urine and convulsions. It occurs where the blood sugar is reading higher than 600 mg/dL; the blood sugar meter may not provide an accurate reading at this level or it may just read "high". Hyperglycemic Hyperosmolar Nonketotic Syndrome is caused by very-high blood sugar that

turns blood thick and syrupy. It tends to be more common in older people with Type 2 Diabetes, and it is often preceded by an illness or infection. Call your Doctor or seek immediate medical care if you have signs or symptoms of this condition.

5.8.2 High Blood Sugar (Hyperglycemia): Of note, a number of factors are responsible for rise in blood sugar, including eating too much, being sick or not taking enough glucose-lowering medication, so, it is desirable to be on the lookout for signs and symptoms of high blood sugar such as— frequent urination, increased thirst, dry mouth, blurred vision, fatigue and nausea.

5.8.3 Increased Ketones In Your Urine (Diabetic Ketoacidosis): Toxic acids known as ketones are produced where your cells are starved for energy, ultimately causing your body to begin to break down fat. It is quite common in people with Type 1 Diabetes. So it is desirable to be on the lookout for thirst or a very dry mouth, frequent urination, vomiting, shortness of breath, fatigue and fruity-smelling breath, to promptly request for emergency care.

5.8.4 Low Blood Sugar (Hypoglycemia): Low blood sugar occurs when the blood sugar level drops below the target range, which could be as a result of skipping a meal, unintentionally taking more medication than usual or getting more physical activity than normal. Notable signs and symptoms of low blood sugar are — sweating, heart palpitations, slurred speech, shakiness, weakness, hunger, irritability, dizziness, headache, drowsiness and confusion. When the aforelisted occur, then try to drink or eat something that will quickly raise your blood sugar level — fruit juice, glucose tablets, hard candy, regular (not diet) soda or another source of sugar. Thereafter, test your blood in 15 minutes to be sure your blood glucose levels have normalized. If you do not get a positive result, treat again and retest in another 15 minutes. If you lose consciousness, a family member or close contact may need to give you an emergency injection of glucagon, which is a hormone that stimulates the release of sugar into the blood.

5.9 When to Consider Bariatric Surgery to Treat Type 2 Diabetes

Major improvements in blood sugar levels are often seen in people with Type 2 Diabetes after bariatric surgery, depending on the procedure performed. Of note, Surgeries that bypass a portion of the small intestine have more of an effect on blood sugar levels than do other weight-loss surgeries. Thus, for Type 2 Diabetes patients whose Body Mass Index (BMI) is greater than 35, you may be a candidate for weight-loss surgery (bariatric surgery) since bariatric surgery is an option for some people with diabetes who are obese and cannot lose weight through diet changes.

However some drawbacks for such surgeries include risk of death and long-term complications may include nutritional deficiencies and osteoporosis. Though it is proven that compared with the medication-only group, people who underwent the surgeries also saw greater reductions in heart disease risk and medication use, as well as an improved quality of life.

Nonetheless, due to the cost and risks, bariatric surgery is usually considered as an option only after less invasive treatments fail.